Menopause Made Easy

Delicious Recipes to Help You Shine

Jasmine Scott

Table Of Contents

Introduction

Has the word "menopause" started to feel like a bit of a buzzkill? Maybe it conjures images of hot flashes, mood swings, and the end of your prime. But what if we told you it could be a time of incredible transformation, a chance to rediscover yourself and embrace a radiant new chapter?

This book is your guide to navigating menopause with a smile – and a delicious plate in hand. We'll shed light on the hormonal changes happening inside you, but we'll also focus on the positive: how to nourish your body for optimal health and well-being.

Forget bland and restrictive diets. Here, you'll find a treasure trove of mouthwatering recipes designed to fuel your energy, manage symptoms, and leave you feeling fantastic. We'll delve into the power of food to balance your hormones, boost your mood, and keep you glowing from within.

So ditch the negativity and get ready to shine. Menopause Made Easy is your invitation to a vibrant journey filled with delicious food, self-care tips, and a celebration of you!

Chapter 1: Welcome to Your Radiant Menopause

Have you ever noticed a small shift? Perhaps it's a random hot flash during a meeting, a challenge to sleep through the night, or a new wrinkle you swear didn't there yesterday. These are the murmurs of a normal transition called menopause. But instead of being concerned, let's reframe the story. Menopause is not the end; it is a lovely new beginning, an opportunity to prioritize your well-being and embark on a brilliant new chapter.

This book is your compass, leading you through the thrilling but often perplexing world of menopause. We'll address misconceptions and misunderstandings, replacing them with evidence-based knowledge and actionable tactics. But, most significantly, we'll commemorate this transforming period with an emphasis on self-care, beginning with the delectable power of food.

Menopause is a natural life stage and not a disease.

Menopause is just the permanent termination of menstruation. It happens when your ovaries progressively cease releasing eggs and estrogen, an important reproductive hormone. This normal decrease often occurs between the ages of 45 and 55, however it might vary.

Menopause signifies the end of your reproductive years, but it is important to recognize that it is not an illness. It's a biological milestone, much like puberty. However, the hormonal changes that occur at this period might induce a range of symptoms, including:

- Hot flushes and nocturnal sweats.
- Vaginal dryness and discomfort.
- Problems sleeping
- Mood swings, irritation
- changes in weight and metabolism
- Lower libido
- difficulty focusing

Understanding the Symphony of Hormone

Our bodies function like sophisticated orchestras, with hormones serving as conductors. Estrogen, progesterone, and testosterone are essential for controlling your menstrual cycle, bone health, mood, and metabolism. During menopause, estrogen production drops considerably, disturbing the delicate hormonal balance. This explains why you may encounter some of the symptoms listed above.

However, it is crucial to realize that each woman's menopausal experience is distinct. Some women have few symptoms, while others encounter a more difficult path. The intensity and length of symptoms may be influenced by a variety of variables, including your general health, genetics, and lifestyle habits.

Accepting the Power of Positive Thinking

Our internal story has a big influence on how we experience menopause. Instead of fearing the changes, let's modify our mindset. Menopause may be seen as a chance for personal development and self-discovery. It's time to put your health first, pursue new hobbies, and rediscover the vibrant woman you are.

Focus on the positives:

Freedom from menstrual pains, leaks, and PMS!

- Increased self-awareness: This is an opportunity to listen to your body's wants and desires.
- Greater emotional clarity: Although estrogen variations might cause mood swings during perimenopause (the years before menopause), some women report feeling more emotionally stable following menopause.
- A opportunity for reinvention: Now is the time to try new hobbies, travel, or pursue interests that you may have put on hold.

Food as Your Ally: Nourish Your Body During Change

What you eat may have a big influence on your health throughout menopause. Food is more than simply nutrition; it is a potent medication that may help you control symptoms, improve your mood, and stay active.

In the next chapters, we'll look at food science and how certain dietary choices might improve your menopausal symptoms. We'll investigate:

- **The power of phytoestrogens**: These plant-based substances mimic the actions of estrogen in the body, possibly reducing hot flashes and other symptoms.
- Gut health: A healthy gut microbiota has been related to enhanced mood control, immunity, and general well-being.

The benefits of anti-inflammatory foods: Chronic inflammation might exacerbate menopausal symptoms. We'll look at delectable meals that use anti-inflammatory components. Essential nutrients for a radiant you: We'll look at the vitamins, minerals, and healthy fats that are essential for keeping strong bones, beautiful skin, and high energy levels throughout menopause.

This journey is yours to own.

Menopause is a unique experience for each woman. Accept the changes, cherish your strengths, and let this book be your guide. With a happy attitude, nutritious dietary choices, and the correct self-care practices, you can face menopause with grace and shine brighter than ever.

So grab your favorite nutritious snack, relax down, and prepare for a delightful and inspiring adventure through menopause. Let us make it a moment of change, not restriction. It's time to change the narrative and celebrate your bright menopause!

Chapter 2: Understanding Your Changing Body—A Symphony of Hormones

Menopause. Some ladies have chills down their spines just hearing the term. It is often represented as a period of abrupt deterioration, a one-way ticket to a world of hot flashes and amnesia. But what if we told you there's another tale to tell?

Menopause is a normal phase that alters your hormonal symphony. Your body is going through a hormonal rebalancing process, similar to how an orchestra conductor alters the pace and loudness of various instruments to produce a new tune. Understanding these changes and their consequences will allow you to traverse this time with grace and awareness.

The Estrogen Equation:

Estrogen, the principal female sex hormone, is a key player in your body's symphony. It affects everything from your menstrual cycle to bone health, emotional management, and skin suppleness. During menopause, estrogen production in the ovaries begins to drop. This drop may set off a series of changes, some slight, others more evident.

Hot flashes and night sweats:

Hot flashes are one of the most prevalent menopausal problems. A rapid burst of heat rushes over your body, typically accompanied by perspiration, flushed skin, and a beating heart. These incidents may be bothersome and unpleasant, but determining the source can be beneficial. The hypothalamus, a region of the brain that controls body temperature, is affected by the drop in estrogen. Misinterpreting signals causes a reaction as if your body is warming, resulting in the typical hot flash. Night sweats are a similar phenomena that may disturb sleep and leave you feeling fatigued.

Beyond The Heat:

The hormonal change might also emerge in other ways. You may notice changes in your sleep habits, such as difficulty falling asleep or staying asleep all night. Reduced estrogen levels may also cause vaginal dryness and pain during intercourse, which can have an influence on your sexual health. Mood swings, impatience, and even brain fog are not unusual, since estrogen regulates neurotransmitters that influence mood and memory.

It's not all downhill.

While certain symptoms may be irritating, it is important to remember that menopause is not an illness. It's a natural part of life, and with the appropriate attitude, you can adapt and prosper. The good news is that the decrease in estrogen is not the only hormonal change occurring. Androgens, a class of hormones often associated with men, also have a function in the female body. Although their levels drop significantly throughout menopause, they may still help to maintain libido and muscular mass.

The significance of individuality:

Menopause is experienced differently by each woman. The degree and kind of symptoms you encounter will be determined by your specific hormone profile, general health, and lifestyle. Some women pass through menopause with little disturbance, while others experience a more difficult path. There is no one "normal" experience, so listen to your body and get help if necessary.

Knowledge is power.

Understanding the hormonal changes that occur during menopause allows you to make educated decisions about treating your symptoms. In the next chapters, we will look at how dietary changes may have a substantial influence on your health. We'll look at particular foods and components that may help relieve hot flashes, enhance sleep quality, and boost your mental wellness. By supporting your body with the appropriate nutrients, you can take an active role in your own health and turn the menopausal journey into a good one.

Remember: you are not alone in this. Millions of women worldwide experience menopause, and there are several tools available to help you. Consult your doctor, connect with other women going through similar situations, and embrace the information that comes with this stage in your life. Menopause is an opportunity to rewrite the script, prioritize self-care, and find new levels of strength and resilience.

Chapter 3: Shine from Within: Adopting a Balanced Diet

Menopause causes a substantial change in your hormonal environment. Estrogen and progesterone, the hormones that traditionally controlled your menstrual cycle, have taken a backseat. This hormonal ebb and flow may cause a slew of symptoms, including hot flashes, nocturnal sweats, weight gain, and exhaustion. But do not be afraid! Food, the fuel that keeps your body going, may be a valuable ally in negotiating these changes.

In this chapter, we'll look at how adopting a balanced diet may be a game changer during menopause. We'll look at the science of food and how it affects your hormones, reveal crucial dietary guidelines, and highlight the advantages of certain items you should integrate into your regular meals.

Food and Hormones: A Delicate Dance.
During menopause, falling estrogen levels may disrupt your metabolism and cause weight gain, especially around the abdomen. This is

because estrogen regulates fat accumulation and use. Furthermore, it may impair insulin sensitivity, making it more difficult for your body to control blood sugar levels.

But there's good news: certain foods may work as natural hormone controllers. Let's look at some significant players:

- Phytoestrogens: Plant-derived chemicals that mimic the actions of estrogen in the body. Flaxseed, lentils, chickpeas, soybeans, and tofu are all excellent sources.
- Cruciferous Vegetables: Broccoli, cauliflower, Brussels sprouts, and kale are high in indoles, which help your body utilize estrogen more effectively.
- Healthy Fats: Omega-3 fatty acids, found in fatty fish such as salmon, sardines, and mackerel, may help decrease inflammation and enhance mood, which are major concerns during menopause. Nuts, seeds, and avocados are all good sources of healthful fat.

Diet Strategies for a Radiant You

Now that we've established the link between food and hormones, let's apply this understanding to practical dietary strategies:

- Prioritize Whole Foods: Avoid processed foods that include harmful fats, refined sugars, and artificial substances. Consume entire, unprocessed foods such as fruits, vegetables, whole grains, lean proteins, and healthy fats. These give necessary nutrients to fuel your body and maintain hormonal equilibrium.
- Embrace Fiber: Fiber is your buddy throughout the menopause. It keeps you feeling fuller for longer, helps with digestion, and regulates blood sugar levels. Aim for at least 25–35 grams of fiber every day. Consume plenty of fruits and vegetables, whole grains like brown rice and quinoa, and legumes such as beans and lentils.
- Limit Added Sugars: Refined sugars may aggravate hot flashes and cause weight gain. Choose natural sweeteners such as fruit or a sprinkling of honey. Be aware of

the hidden sugars in processed meals, sauces, and sugary beverages.

- Stay Hydrated: Dehydration may produce symptoms such as hot flushes and exhaustion. Aim for eight glasses of water every day. Refreshing choices include herbal teas and fruit and vegetable-infused water.

- Calcium and Vitamin D Powerhouse: As estrogen levels decline throughout menopause, bone health becomes a top issue. Consume calcium-rich foods such as dairy products, leafy greens, fortified plant-based milks, and tofu. Vitamin D promotes calcium absorption, so include fatty fish and sunlight (in moderation) in your daily routine.

Insights into Superfood Ingredients

Now that we've established a strong nutritional basis, let's look at some superstar ingredients that can elevate your meals to the next level:

- Berries, which are high in antioxidants and phytoestrogens, may help decrease inflammation and maintain hormonal balance. Examples include blueberries, raspberries, and strawberries.

- Flaxseeds: These small seeds are a triple threat, including fiber, omega-3 fatty acids, and lignans, a phytoestrogen. Grind them fresh and sprinkle over salads, yogurt, or cereal.
- Greek yogurt, a high-protein and calcium-rich food, may help regulate appetite and promote bone health. Choose simple varieties and garnish with fruits, nuts, or a drizzle of honey.
- Salmon: This omega-3 fatty acid superfood may boost mood, lower inflammation, and promote heart health. Enjoy it roasted, grilled, or poached.
- Quinoa is a complete protein grain high in fiber, iron, and magnesium, all of which are vital elements during menopause. Use it as the foundation for bowls, salads, or as a side dish.

Remember that a balanced diet is not about restriction; it is about variety and nutrition. Experiment with various tastes and textures until you discover nutritious meals you like.

This chapter is just the beginning of your delectable adventure through menopause. In the next chapter, we'll delve into a treasure mine of dishes that embrace these nutritional guidelines while tantalizing your taste senses. So be ready to cook up a storm and embrace your glowing, healthy self!

Chapter 4: Delicious Recipes for Everyday

Menopause does not have to mean compromising taste or giving up your favorite foods. This chapter will show you how to prepare tasty and nutritious meals that will help you stay healthy throughout this shift. We'll concentrate on combining crucial components that alleviate typical menopausal symptoms while delighting your taste buds.

Build a Balanced Plate:

Before we get into recipes, let's look at the components of a menopause-friendly diet. Imagine dividing your plate into three sections:

- Half filled with bright veggies and fruits: These brilliant powerhouses are high in antioxidants that combat inflammation and promote heart health, both of which are important during menopause. Consider leafy greens, berries, bell peppers, and sweet potatoes; the rainbow is your guide!

- One-quarter full of lean protein: Protein is necessary for maintaining muscular mass, which might decrease after menopause. Fish, chicken, beans, lentils, and tofu are excellent sources of energy and satisfaction.

- The remaining quarter should be packed with good grains or healthy fats, such as whole wheat bread, brown rice, quinoa, or avocado or olive oil. These give long-lasting energy and ensure proper hormone balance.

Now, let's apply these concepts to some great meals!

Breakfast Powerhouse:

- Scrambled Eggs with Spinach and Smoked Salmon: This protein-rich meal is ideal for controlling hot flashes. Eggs have high levels of vitamin D, which may help regulate body temperature. Spinach contains iron, which is necessary for energy generation, while smoked salmon has healthful omega-3 fatty acids that combat inflammation. Scramble eggs with chopped spinach, then top with flaky smoked salmon. Finally, sprinkle with minced chives.

Lunch Time Delight:

- Mediterranean Chickpea Salad with Pita Bread: This fiber-rich salad is ideal for keeping you full and content. Chickpeas are a plant-based protein powerhouse, while chopped veggies such as cucumber, tomatoes, and red onion provide a crisp crunch. Toss everything with a delicious dressing of olive oil, lemon juice, oregano, and a dash of garlic powder. Serve with whole wheat pita bread for dipping.

Dinner Time Feast:

- Salmon with Roasted Vegetables and Quinoa: This heart-healthy recipe is full of taste and nutrition. Salmon has high levels of omega-3 fatty acids, which may aid with mood fluctuations and cognitive performance. Roast broccoli, Brussels sprouts, and sweet potato cubes in olive oil, salt, and pepper. Pan-sear salmon fillets seasoned with lemon pepper and serve over roasted veggies on a bed of fluffy quinoa.

Sweet Treat Satisfaction:

- Dark Chocolate Avocado Mousse: Want something sweet? Look no further! This velvety mousse will satisfy your sweet taste while providing health advantages. Avocados are abundant in healthy fats that help regulate mood, while dark chocolate (70% cacao or higher) contains antioxidants and mood-boosting chemicals. Blend the ripe avocado, unsweetened cocoa powder, honey, and almond milk until creamy. Add a sprinkling of chocolate nibs for texture.

Snacks on the go:

Don't allow hungry sensations lead to poor decisions. Keep these nutritious snacks on hand.

- Greek yogurt with berries and honey contains protein and calcium, which promotes bone health.
- A handful of almonds and dried cranberries provides a pleasing balance of protein, healthy fats, and antioxidants.
- Carrot sticks and hummus are a traditional fiber-rich combination that helps regulate blood sugar levels.

Remember:

Here are just a few samples to get you started. Experiment with various tastes and ingredients to create meals that you like. Don't be hesitant to change portion sizes depending on your specific requirements and exercise level.

Spice it up!

Adding certain herbs and spices may enrich your meals and may provide extra health benefits:

- Ginger is known for its anti-inflammatory effects, which may assist with hot flashes and nausea. Try mixing it into stir-fries or marinades.

- Turmeric: Another powerful anti-inflammatory, turmeric may aid with joint pain and mood. Use ground turmeric in recipes or sprinkle it over roasted veggies.
- Flaxseed is high in omega-3 fatty acids and fiber, which may help with heart health and digestion. Grind flaxseeds and mix them into smoothies, porridge, or baked goods.

Embrace the journey

Cooking is a method of self-care. Take the time to relish your meals and enjoy the process of preparing tasty and nutritional recipes that will benefit your health throughout menopause. Remember: food is your buddy. Use it to energize your body, celebrate your health, and radiate from inside!

Chapter 5: Enjoy the Journey: Food, Fun, and Celebrating Yourself

Menopause is a big milestone, a time to reflect on the magnificent trip your body has brought you on. It's also an opportunity to welcome a new chapter full with possibilities. But, let's be honest, dealing with hormone shifts and their consequences on your physical and mental health may be daunting at times.

This chapter goes beyond the plate and delves into the world of holistic wellbeing. We'll look at how diet, together with stress management, relaxation methods, and regular exercise, may help you live a vibrant and meaningful life throughout and beyond menopause.

Food for your mind, body, and soul

The link between diet and mood is apparent. During menopause, hormonal fluctuations may have an influence on your mental state, causing anxiety, irritation, and even sadness. The good news is that food choices may have a substantial impact on your mental well-being.

- Focus on Mood-Boosting Foods: Eat foods high in omega-3 fatty acids, such as salmon, flaxseeds, and walnuts. These lipids are necessary for brain function and may alleviate symptoms of despair and anxiety.
- Embrace Complex Carbs: Replace refined carbohydrates with complex carbs such as whole grains, sweet potatoes, and quinoa. These give long-lasting energy and help manage blood sugar levels, which might influence mood swings.
- Don't skimp on fruits and vegetables; aim for a rainbow on your plate! Fruits and vegetables are high in vitamins, minerals, and antioxidants, all of which help to reduce inflammation and improve overall health.

Beyond the Kitchen: Promoting Inner Peace

While diet is important, flourishing throughout menopause requires a balanced approach. Here are some ways to nourish your mind and spirit:

- Mindfulness and Meditation: Spend even a few minutes every day doing mindfulness exercises or meditation. These techniques may help you manage stress, concentrate better, and feel calmer.

- Get Moving: Regular physical exercise is an effective stress reliever, improves sleep quality, and boosts mood. Find activities that you love, such as dancing, swimming, brisk walking, or taking a fitness class.

- The Importance of Sleep: Prioritize good sleep. Aim to get 7-8 hours of unbroken sleep each night. Establish a calm nighttime ritual and establish a sleep-promoting atmosphere.

- Connect and Nurture Relationships: Social relationships are critical to emotional well-being. Spend time with loved ones, attend a support group, or catch up with old pals.

- Embrace Self-Care: Don't underestimate the value of treating oneself. Take a soothing bath, have a massage, or engage in a creative pursuit you like. Make time for things that make you happy and leave you feeling revitalized.

We're Celebrating You!

Menopause is not a sickness; it is a normal change. It's time to honor your achievements, knowledge, and strength. Here are some ways to appreciate oneself during this transformational period:

- Revisit Passions: Have you set aside hobbies or interests because of life's demands? Menopause might be an ideal moment to rekindle old hobbies or discover new ones.
- Travel and Explore: Have you always wanted to visit a certain location? Now is the moment to make it happen! Travel can be a transforming experience, expanding your horizons and instilling a feeling of adventure.

- Learn Something New: To keep your mind bright and interested, try a new skill, take a class, or read inspirational literature.
- Embrace Gratitude: Take time every day to recognize the positive things in your life, no matter how large or little. Gratitude is a strong technique for increasing pleasure and well-being.

Remember that you are not alone on this path. Surround yourself with supporting friends, adopt healthy habits, and enjoy the delectable meals in this cookbook. Menopause may be a period of profound self-discovery and an opportunity to live a life that really shines. So, let us raise a fork (filled with something yummy) to you and this wonderful new chapter!

Conclusion

"Menopause Made Easy." We hope you've discovered a treasure trove of delicious recipes that nourish your body and tantalize your taste buds. But more importantly, we trust this book has empowered you to embrace menopause as a chance for transformation and self-discovery.

Remember, menopause is not the end – it's a beautiful new beginning. With a focus on nourishing your body with delicious, wholesome foods, prioritizing self-care practices, and celebrating your amazing self, you can navigate this transition with grace and confidence.

As you embark on this radiant new chapter, keep these words close to your heart: You are strong, you are capable, and you are worthy. Keep shining your light, and never stop celebrating the incredible woman you are!